Noninvasive Breast Cancer

LEARNING that you have cancer can be overwhelming.

The goal of this book is to help you get the best care. It presents which tests and treatments are recommended by experts in breast cancer.

The National Comprehensive Cancer Network® (NCCN®) is a not-for-profit alliance of 27 of the world's leading cancer centers. Experts from NCCN have written treatment guidelines for doctors who treat breast cancer. These treatment guidelines suggest what the best practice is for cancer care. The information in this patient book is based on the guidelines written for doctors.

This book focuses on the treatment of noninvasive breast cancer. Key points of the book are summarized in the related NCCN Quick Guide™. NCCN also offers patient resources on invasive and metastatic breast cancer, ovarian cancer, sarcoma, lymphomas, and other cancer types. Visit NCCN.org/patients for the full library of patient books, summaries, and other resources.

About

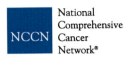

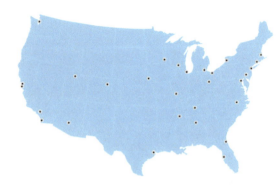

These patient guidelines for cancer care are produced by the National Comprehensive Cancer Network® (NCCN®).

The mission of NCCN is to improve cancer care so people can live better lives. At the core of NCCN are the NCCN Clinical Practice Guidelines in Oncology (NCCN Guidelines®). NCCN Guidelines® contain information to help health care workers plan the best cancer care. They list options for cancer care that are most likely to have the best results. The NCCN Guidelines for Patients® present the information from the NCCN Guidelines in an easy-to-learn format.

Panels of experts create the NCCN Guidelines. Most of the experts are from NCCN Member Institutions. Their areas of expertise are diverse. Many panels also include a patient advocate. Recommendations in the NCCN Guidelines are based on clinical trials and the experience of the panelists. The NCCN Guidelines are updated at least once a year. When funded, the patient books are updated to reflect the most recent version of the NCCN Guidelines for doctors.

For more information about the NCCN Guidelines, visit NCCN.org/clinical.asp.

Dorothy A. Shead, MS *Director, Patient Information Operations*	Laura J. Hanisch, PsyD *Medical Writer/Patient Information Specialist*	Erin Vidic, MA *Medical Writer*
	Alycia Corrigan *Medical Writer*	Rachael Clarke *Guidelines Data and Layout Coordinator*

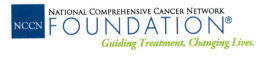

NCCN Foundation was founded by NCCN to raise funds for patient education based on the NCCN Guidelines. NCCN Foundation offers guidance to people with cancer and their caregivers at every step of their cancer journey. This is done by sharing key information from leading cancer experts. This information can be found in a library of NCCN Guidelines for Patients® and other patient education resources. NCCN Foundation is also committed to advancing cancer treatment by funding the nation's promising doctors at the center of cancer research, education, and progress of cancer therapies.

For more information about NCCN Foundation, visit NCCNFoundation.org.

© 2018 National Comprehensive Cancer Network, Inc. Based on the NCCN Clinical Practice Guidelines in Oncology (NCCN Guidelines®) Breast Cancer (Version 1.2018). Posted 06/07/2018.

All rights reserved. NCCN Guidelines for Patients® and illustrations herein may not be reproduced in any form for any purpose without the express written permission of NCCN. No one, including doctors or patients, may use the NCCN Guidelines for Patients® for any commercial purpose and may not claim, represent, or imply that the NCCN Guidelines for Patients® that has been modified in any manner is derived from, based on, related to or arises out of the NCCN Guidelines for Patients®. The NCCN Guidelines are a work in progress that may be redefined as often as new significant data become available. NCCN makes no warranties of any kind whatsoever regarding its content, use, or application and disclaims any responsibility for its application or use in any way.

National Comprehensive Cancer Network (NCCN) • 275 Commerce Drive, Suite 300 • Fort Washington, PA 19034 • 215.690.0300

Cover photo: Copyright ©2018 Young Survival Coalition (YSC).

Supporters

Endorsed by

Breast Cancer Alliance
Receiving a cancer diagnosis can be overwhelming, both for the patient and their family. We support the NCCN guidelines for breast cancer with the knowledge that these tools will help to equip patients with many of the educational resources, and answers to questions, they may seek.
breastcanceralliance.org

FORCE: Facing Our Risk of Cancer Empowered
As the nation's leading organization serving the hereditary breast and ovarian cancer community, FORCE is pleased to endorse the NCCN Guidelines for Patients on breast cancer. This guide provides valuable, evidence-based, expert-reviewed information on the standard of care, empowering patients to make informed decisions about their treatment.
www.facingourrisk.org

Living Beyond Breast Cancer
Receiving a diagnosis of breast cancer is overwhelming. Having trusted information is essential to help understand one's particular diagnosis and treatment options. The information found in the NCCN Guidelines for Patients: Breast Cancer is accessible, accurate, and will help every step of the way—from the moment of diagnosis through treatment. People can use the NCCN Guidelines for Patients: Breast Cancer to become an informed partner in their own care. lbbc.org

Sharsharet
Sharsheret is proud to endorse this important resource, the NCCN Guidelines for Patients: Breast Cancer. With this critical tool in hand, women nationwide have the knowledge they need to partner with their healthcare team to navigate the often complicated world of breast cancer care and make informed treatment decisions. www.sharsheret.org

Young Survival Coalition (YSC)
Young Survival Coalition (YSC) is pleased to endorse the NCCN Guidelines for Patients: Breast Cancer as an invaluable resource for young women diagnosed with breast cancer and their co-survivors. This in-depth, illustrated series clearly explains what breast cancer is, how it is treated and what patients can expect on the journey ahead.
youngsurvival.org

With generous support from

In Honor of Janet M. Smedley (Breast Cancer Survivor).
Special thanks to the members and staff of Orangetheory Fitness, Gwynedd PA for their generous donation.

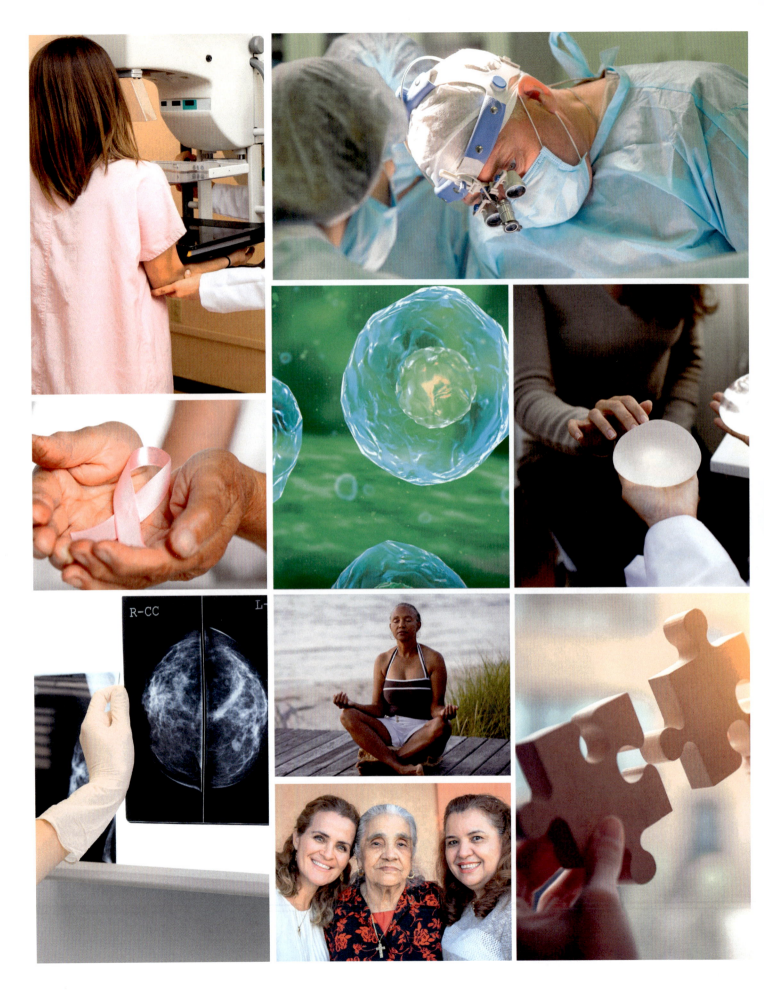

Noninvasive Breast Cancer

Contents

6   How to use this book

7   Part 1
Breast cancer basics
Explains breast cancer and staging.

14   Part 2
Treatment guide:
Paget disease
Presents treatment options for breast cancer confined to the nipple-areola complex.

20   Part 3
Treatment guide:
DCIS
Presents treatment options for breast cancer confined to the ducts.

28   Part 4
Treatment guide:
Breast reconstruction
Presents methods to rebuild breasts after they are removed.

31   Part 5
Making treatment decisions
Offers tips for choosing the best treatment.

40   Dictionary

42   Acronyms

43   NCCN Panel Members for Breast Cancer

44   NCCN Member Institutions

46   Index

How to use this book

Who should read this book?

Treatment for noninvasive breast cancers is the focus of this book. Noninvasive means the cancer hasn't entered into the fatty part of the breast. The cancer is in either the ducts, or nipple and areola. They are also called breast carcinoma in situ and stage 0 breast cancer.

Almost all breast cancers occur in women. As such, this book is written with women in mind. However, for noninvasive breast cancer, men receive the same treatment as women.

Patients and those who support them—caregivers, family, and friends—may find this book helpful. It is a good starting point to learn what your options may be.

Are the book chapters in a certain order?

Early chapters explain concepts that are repeated in later chapters. **Part 1** explains what breast cancer is. Read **Part 2** to learn what health care is advised for Paget disease. Treatment for DCIS is covered in **Part 3**. Read **Part 4** to learn some methods of breast reconstruction after breast cancer surgery. Tips for making treatment decisions are presented in **Part 5**.

Does this book include all options?

This book includes treatment options for most people. Your treatment team can point out what applies to you. They can also give you more information. While reading, make a list of questions to ask your doctors.

The treatment options are based on science and the experience of NCCN experts. However, their recommendations may not be right for you. Your doctors may suggest other options based on your health and other factors. If other options are given, ask your treatment team questions.

Help! What do the words mean?

In this book, many medical words are included. These are words that your treatment team may say to you. Most of these words may be new to you. It may be a lot to learn.

Don't be discouraged as you read. Keep reading and review the information. Ask your treatment team to explain a word or phrase that you do not understand.

Words that you may not know are defined in the text or in the *Dictionary*. *Acronyms* are also defined when first used and in the *Glossary*. Acronyms are short words formed from the first letters of several words. One example is DNA for **d**eoxyribo**n**ucleic **a**cid.

1
Breast cancer basics

- 8   Women's breasts
- 10   A disease of cells
- 10   Cancer's threat
- 12   Cancer stages
- 13   Review

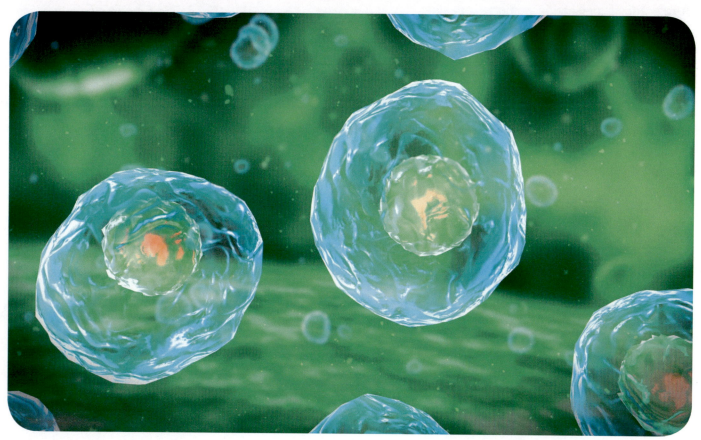

1 Breast cancer basics | Women's breasts

You've learned that you have breast cancer. It's common to feel shocked and confused. This chapter reviews some basics that may help you learn about breast cancer.

Women's breasts

Before learning about breast cancer, it is helpful to know about breasts. The ring of darker breast skin is called the areola. The raised tip within the areola is called the nipple. The nipple-areola complex is a term that refers to both parts.

Under the nipple are ducts within a fatty tissue called stroma. During puberty, the breasts of girls change a lot. The stroma increases. The ducts grow and branch out into the stroma. At the end of the ducts, millions of small sacs called lobules form. **See Figure 1** for a look inside women's breasts.

Lymph is a clear fluid that gives cells water and food. It also helps to fight germs. Lymph drains from breast tissue into vessels within the stroma. **See Figure 2**.

From the breast, lymph travels to the breast's lymph nodes. Lymph nodes are small structures that remove germs from lymph. Most of your breast's lymph nodes are in your armpit. Nodes near the armpit are called axillary lymph nodes.

1 Breast cancer basics | Women's breasts

Figure 1
Inside of breasts

Inside of women's breasts are millions of lobules. Lobules form breast milk after a baby is born. Breast milk drains from the lobules into ducts that carry the milk to the nipple. Around the lobules and ducts is soft tissue called stroma.

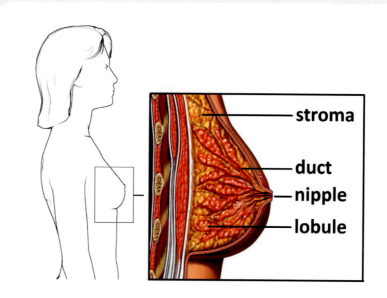

Figure 2
Breast lymph vessels and nodes

Lymph is a clear fluid that gives cells water and food. It drains from breast tissue into lymph vessels within the stroma. It then travels to the breast's lymph nodes. Most of the breast's lymph nodes are near the armpit. These nodes are called axillary lymph nodes.

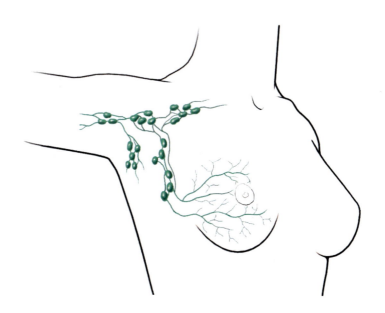

1 Breast cancer basics | A disease of cells | Cancer's threat

A disease of cells

Your body is made of trillions of cells. Cancer is a disease of cells. Each type of cancer is named after the cell from which it derived. Breast cancer is a cancer of breast cells.

Almost all breast cancers are carcinomas. Carcinomas are cancers of cells that line the inner or outer surfaces of the body. Most breast cancers are derived from cells that line the ducts.

Mutations

Cells have a control center called the nucleus. Within the nucleus are chromosomes. Chromosomes are long strands of DNA (**d**eoxyribo**n**ucleic **a**cid) that are tightly wrapped around proteins. **See Figure 3**. Within DNA are coded instructions for building new cells and controlling how cells behave. These instructions are called genes.

There can be abnormal changes in genes called mutations. Some types of mutations that are linked to cancer are present in all cells. Other mutations are present only in cancer cells. Mutations cause cancer cells to not behave like normal cells. They sometimes cause cancer cells to look very different from normal cells.

Cancer's threat

When needed, normal cells grow and then divide to form new cells. When old or damaged, they die as shown in **Figure 4**. Normal cells also stay in place. Cancer cells don't behave like normal cells. Cancer cells differ from normal cells in three key ways.

Mass of cells

Cancer cells make new cells that aren't needed. They don't die quickly when old or damaged. Over time, cancer cells form a mass called the primary tumor.

Invasion

Cancer cells can grow into surrounding tissues. If not treated, the primary tumor can grow through a duct or lobule into the stroma. Breast cancers that haven't grown into the stroma are called "noninvasive." Breast cancers that have grown into the stroma are called "invasive."

Metastasis

Third, unlike normal cells, cancer cells can leave the breast. This process is called metastasis. In this process, cancer cells break away from the tumor and merge with blood or lymph. Then, the cancer cells travel through blood or lymph vessels to other sites. Once in other sites, cancer cells may form secondary tumors. Over time, major health problems can occur.

1 Breast cancer basics | Cancer's threat

**Figure 3
Genetic material in cells**

Most human cells contain a plan called the "blueprint of life." It is a plan for how our bodies are made and work. It is found inside of chromosomes. Chromosomes are long strands of DNA that are tightly wrapped around proteins. Genes are small pieces of DNA. Humans have about 20,000 to 25,000 genes.

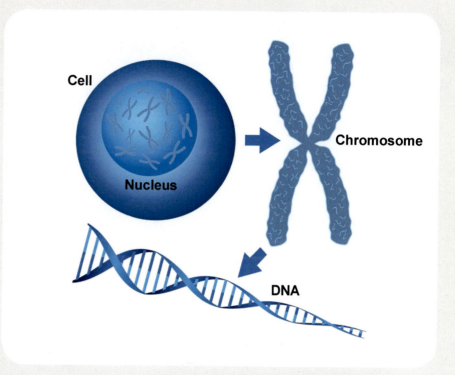

**Figure 4
Normal cell growth vs. cancer cell growth**

Normal cells increase in number when they are needed. They also die when old or damaged. In contrast, cancer cells quickly make new cells and live longer.

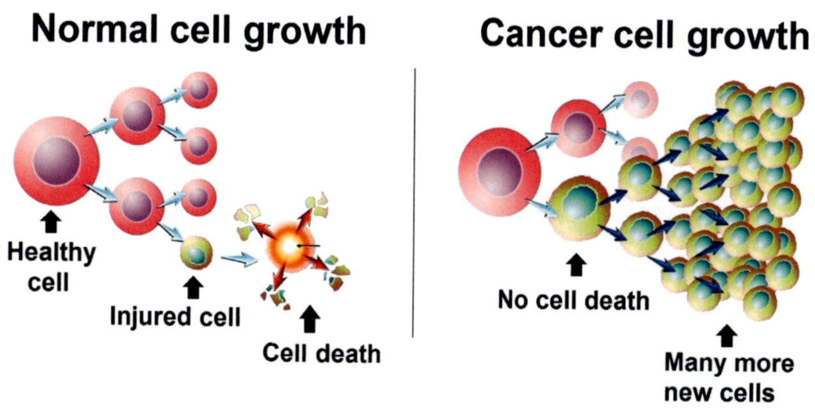

Illustration Copyright © 2018 Nucleus Medical Media, All rights reserved. www.nucleusinc.com

1 Breast cancer basics | Cancer stages

Cancer stages

A cancer stage is a rating of the cancer based on test results. Your doctor uses it for many things. It is used to assess the outlook of the cancer (prognosis). It is used to plan treatment. It is also used for research.

Cancer staging is often done twice. The rating before any treatment is called the clinical stage. The rating after receiving only surgery is called the pathologic stage.

Staging system
The AJCC (**A**merican **J**oint **C**ommittee on **C**ancer) staging system is used to stage breast cancer. In the past, breast cancer was staged only based on its extent in the body. The current system has staging charts that are based on extent as well as other factors.

TNM scores
Three scores are used to describe the extent of the cancer. The T score describes the growth of the primary tumor. The N score describes cancer growth within nearby lymph nodes. Nearby nodes are on the same side of the chest as the breast tumor. The M score tells if the cancer has spread to distant sites.

Numbered stages
The TNM scores and other factors are used to stage cancer. The stages of breast cancer are labeled by numbers. They range from stage 0 to stage 4. Doctors write these stages in Roman numbers—stage 0, stage I, stage II, stage III, and stage IV.

Stage 0
Noninvasive breast cancers are rated stage 0. These cancers have not grown into the stroma. They have not spread to other tissues. There are two types.

> - DCIS (**d**uctal **c**arcinoma **in** **s**itu) is only in the breast ducts.

> - Paget disease of the nipple is only in the nipple and areola.

Stages I–III
Invasive breast cancers are rated stage I, II, or III. These cancers have grown into the stroma or breast skin. Some have spread to nearby sites. None have spread to distant parts of the body.

Stage IV
Metastatic breast cancers have spread to distant sites. Stage IV is metastatic cancer that was present at diagnosis. Over time, other stages of breast cancer sometimes metastasize.

1 Breast cancer basics | Review

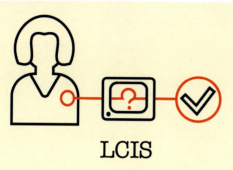

LCIS

LCIS (**l**obular **c**arcinoma **i**n **s**itu) used to be rated as stage 0. However, it isn't cancer. It is an abnormal cell growth confined to the lobules. As such, it is no longer included in the staging system.

LCIS is one of many factors that increases your chance for breast cancer. Another factor is your family history. Your doctor will tell you what your chance of breast cancer is.

Risk-reduction treatment is advised for some women. This treatment may include living a healthier lifestyle. You may be prescribed drugs that stop cancer growth caused by hormones. Women at high risk for breast cancer may have both breasts removed.

Breast cancer screening is advised for all women who've had LCIS. The aim of screening is to find cancer early when treatment will work best. Your doctor will create a screening plan that is right for you.

Review

- Inside of women's breasts are lobules, ducts, and stroma. Lobules are structures that make breast milk. Ducts carry breast milk from the lobules to the nipple. Stroma is a soft tissue that surrounds the lobules and ducts.

- Breast cancer often starts in the ducts and then spreads into the stroma.

- Breast cancer that has not grown into the stroma is called noninvasive.

- Once in the stroma, breast cancer can spread through lymph or blood to other sites.

- Noninvasive breast cancers are rated stage 0. There are two types. DCIS is confined to the ducts. Paget disease is confined to the nipple and areola.

2 Treatment guide: Paget disease

15 Treatment planning
18 Cancer treatment
18 Risk reduction
19 Follow-up care
19 Review

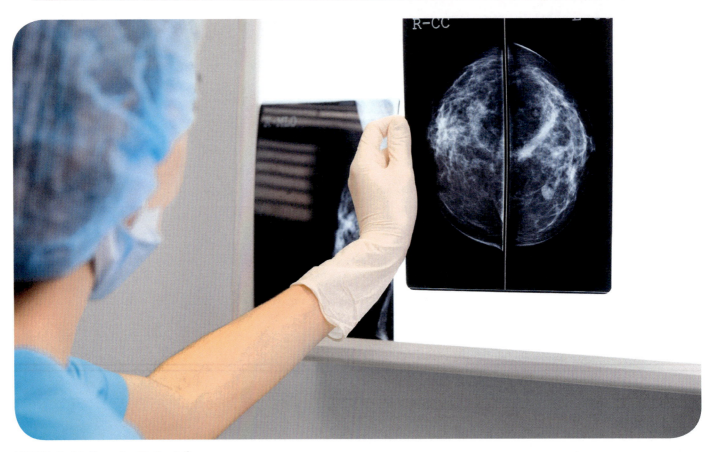

2 Treatment guide: Paget disease | Treatment planning

Paget disease of the nipple is a rare type of breast cancer. This chapter describes the tests for Paget disease. It also presents treatment options for women who only have Paget disease.

Treatment planning

Paget disease is a rare type of breast cancer among women. It occurs even less often in men. Most of the time, Paget disease occurs in only one breast.

Paget disease changes how the nipple feels and looks. Feelings of pain, burning, soreness, and itchiness are common. A nipple may look red, scaly, flaky, or raw. Tiny sores are common. Less commonly, a nipple will bleed or become sunken. Changes to your areola may also occur.

See your doctor if you have symptoms of Paget disease. These symptoms can be caused by other diseases. Your doctor will ask questions about your health history. Be prepared to report the health history of your close blood relatives. If your doctor suspects breast cancer, you will need to receive some tests. These tests are described next.

Clinical breast exam

Your doctor will look closely at and touch your bare breasts. The area around your breasts will also be viewed and touched. Your doctor may want you to sit, stand up, or lie down during the exam. You may feel nervous having your breasts touched. Keep in mind that this exam is quick and provides key information your doctor needs.

Imaging

Imaging tests make pictures of the insides of your body. They are used to find cancer. Your treatment team will tell you how to prepare for these tests. A radiologist is a doctor who's an expert in reading images. He or she will convey the test results to your doctor.

You may need to stop taking some medicines. You may need to stop eating and drinking for a few hours before the scan. Tell your doctors if you get nervous when in small spaces. You may be given a pill to help you relax.

Diagnostic bilateral mammogram

A mammogram is a picture of the insides of your breast. The pictures are made using x-rays. A computer combines the x-rays to make detailed pictures. **See Figure 5**.

Diagnostic mammograms are made with more x-rays than screening mammograms. With more x-rays, tumors can be better seen if present. A bilateral mammogram is a picture of each breast.

Ultrasound

Ultrasound uses sound waves to make pictures. A probe will be held on your bare breast. It may also be placed below your armpit. The picture will be seen on a screen while the probe is in use.

Ultrasound is sometimes used if Paget disease is present. It may be used to further assess a mass. It may also be used to help remove tissue samples for testing.

Breast MRI

If you have Paget disease, you may receive breast MRI (**m**agnetic **r**esonance **i**maging). It is used to

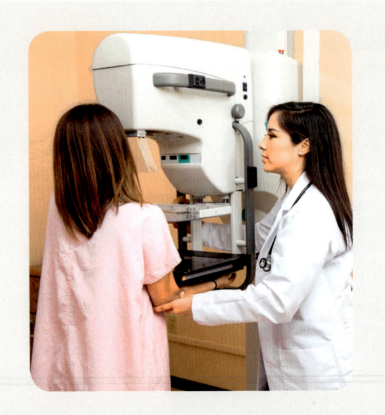

Figure 5
Mammogram

A mammogram is a picture of the insides of your breast. It is produced by an imaging machine. As shown, you will need to stand next to the machine. Your breast will be placed onto a flat surface, called a plate. A second plate will be lowered onto your breast to flatten it. This may be painful but it gets the least fuzzy picture of your breast. A camera attached to the two plates will take pictures.

look for cancer not found on mammogram. It does produce false alarms. So, the tissue that may have cancer should be tested.

This test uses a magnetic field and radio waves to make pictures. Contrast should be used if you've had no prior problems with it. It is a dye that makes the pictures clearer.

You will need to lie face down on a table. The table will have padded openings for your bare breasts. During the scan, the table will move slowly through a machine.

Biopsy

A biopsy is a procedure that removes tissue or fluid samples for testing. It is needed to confirm if cancer cells are present. The samples will be sent to a lab for testing.

Full-thickness skin biopsy

You will need a skin biopsy. There is more than one type. Some types scrape off a little skin from the top skin layer. Other types remove some skin from the top and bottom layers. The types that remove both layers are better for Paget disease.

Common methods include a wedge and punch biopsy. The wedge method uses a sharp knife called a scalpel. Skin samples and maybe ductal cells will be removed. The punch method uses a sharp, hollow cutting device. This device removes small but deep skin samples.

Core biopsy of breast mass

A core biopsy removes tissue samples with a hollow needle. It is advised if there's a mass within the breast. Imaging may be used to guide the needle into the tumor. A stereotactic needle biopsy uses mammography.

Waiting for results is often the hardest part of this journey. I am an overachiever when it comes to thinking about worse case scenarios when I don't have all the information.

– Deb
  Cancer Survivor

Cancer treatment

Almost all people with Paget disease have cancer elsewhere in their breast. If there is invasive cancer, read the *NCCN Guidelines for Patients: Breast Cancer – Invasive*. Read Part 3 in this book to learn the treatment options for Paget disease with DCIS.

Lab tests may have found only Paget disease. This section describes treatment options for you. Treatment options are listed in Guide 1. You may have more than one option for treatment. Read Part 5 to learn tips on making treatment decisions.

Central lumpectomy
The nipple-areola complex is removed during a central lumpectomy. Normal-looking tissue beneath the complex is also removed to try to remove all the cancer. Most of your breast will remain. Read Part 4 to learn about breast reconstruction after lumpectomy.

Total mastectomy
The whole breast is removed during a total mastectomy. Chest muscle is not removed. This operation is also called a simple mastectomy. A skin-sparing mastectomy removes the breast but not the skin. Read Part 5 to learn about methods of breast reconstruction.

Radiation therapy
For breast cancer, radiation therapy uses high-energy x-rays. The x-rays destroy cancer cells that may remain in the breast after lumpectomy. The whole breast should be treated.

Sentinel lymph node biopsy
Sentinel nodes are the first nodes to which lymph travels after leaving the breast. An SLNB (**s**entinel **l**ymph **n**ode **b**iopsy) finds and removes 2 or 3 of these nodes. The nodes are then tested for cancer.

Clinical trial
A clinical trial is a type of research that studies a test or treatment in people. It gives people access to health care that otherwise can't usually be received. Ask your treatment team if there is an open clinical trial that you can join.

Risk reduction

Talk to your doctor about ways to reduce your chance of a second breast cancer. Risk reduction has not been well studied after treatment for Paget disease. However, it has been shown to work well after treatment for DCIS.

There are three ways to reduce your risk. Living a healthier lifestyle may be helpful. A second way is to take prescribed drugs like tamoxifen or letrozole. Women at high risk for breast cancer may have both breasts removed.

Guide 1. Treatment for Paget disease

What are the options?
• Central lumpectomy + radiation therapy
• Total mastectomy ± sentinel lymph node biopsy
• Central lumpectomy ± sentinel lymph node biopsy
• Clinical trial

Follow-up care

Follow-up care is important for your long-term health. It is started after treatment ends. There must be no signs or symptoms of cancer.

Medical history and physical exam
An update of your health history and physical exam are part of follow-up care. Both should be done every 6 to 12 months for 5 years. After 5 years of normal results, these tests are needed once a year.

Mammogram
A mammogram should be done every 12 months. The first one may be received as soon as 6 months after breast-conserving treatment. Mammograms aren't needed if you had both breasts removed to reduce your cancer risk.

Review

- Your doctor may suspect that you have Paget disease of the nipple based on symptoms.

- A clinical breast exam and imaging will be needed to assess for abnormal tissue.

- To confirm if breast cancer is present, samples of tissue must be removed and tested.

- If only Paget disease if present, the nipple-areola complex or whole breast may be removed. You may receive radiation therapy after the nipple-areola complex is removed.

- After cancer treatment, visit your doctor once or twice a year. He or she will assess for any new signs or symptoms of breast cancer.

3 Treatment guide: DCIS

- 21 Treatment planning
- 24 Cancer treatment
- 26 Risk-reduction treatment
- 27 Follow-up care
- 27 Review

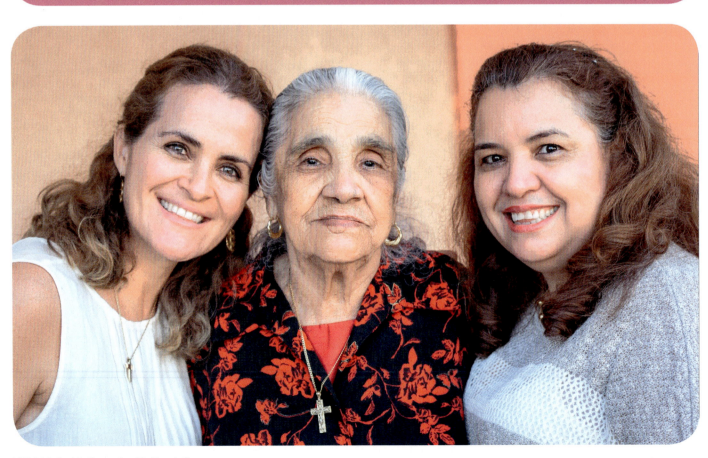

3 Treatment guide: DCIS | Treatment planning

DCIS is a breast cancer that is confined to the ducts. This chapter lists the tests to plan treatment for DCIS. It also presents treatment options on cancer treatment and the next steps of health care.

Treatment planning

Medical history

Your doctor will ask about any health problems and treatment during your lifetime. Be prepared to tell what illnesses and injuries you have had. You will also be asked about health conditions and symptoms. It may help to bring a list of old and new medicines to your doctor's office.

Some cancers and other health problems can run in families. Thus, your doctor will ask about the medical history of your close blood relatives. Such family includes your siblings, parents, and grandparents. Be prepared to tell who has had what diseases and at what ages.

Hereditary breast cancer is due to abnormal genes that were passed down from parent to child. It is not common. About 1 out of 10 breast cancers are hereditary. Read *Genetic counseling* at the end of this section to learn more.

Physical exam

A physical exam is a study of your body. It is done to look for signs of disease. It is also used to help assess what treatments may be options.

To start, your basic body functions will be measured. These functions include your temperature, blood pressure, and pulse and breathing rate. Your weight will also be checked.

Your doctor will listen to your lungs, heart, and gut. He or she will also assess your eyes, skin, nose, ears, and mouth. Parts of your body will be felt. Your doctor will note the size of organs and if they feel soft or hard. Tell your doctor if you feel pain when touched.

Clinical breast exam

Your doctor will look closely at and touch your bare breasts. The area around your breasts will also be viewed and touched. Your doctor may want you to sit, stand up, or lie down during the exam. You may feel nervous having your breasts touched. Keep in mind that this exam is quick and provides key information your doctor needs.

Imaging

Imaging tests make pictures of the insides of your body. They are used to find cancer. Your treatment team will tell you how to prepare for these tests. A radiologist is a doctor who's an expert in reading images. He or she will convey the test results to your doctor.

You may need to stop taking some medicines. You may need to stop eating and drinking for a few hours before the scan. Tell your doctors if you get nervous when in small spaces. You may be given a pill to help you relax.

Diagnostic bilateral mammogram

A mammogram is a picture of the insides of your breast. The pictures are made using x-rays. A computer combines the x-rays to make detailed pictures.

Diagnostic mammograms are made with more x-rays than screening mammograms. With more x-rays, tumors can be better seen if present. A bilateral mammogram includes pictures of both breasts.

3 Treatment guide: DCIS | Treatment planning

You may have had a recent diagnostic bilateral mammogram. If not, it is advised. Results are used to plan treatment.

Breast MRI
Breast MRI is not often used for DCIS. Your doctor may order it if the mammogram is unclear. It may help show the extent of the cancer. It does produce false alarms. Thus, tissue that may have cancer should be tested.

This test uses a magnetic field and radio waves to make pictures. Contrast should be used if you've had no prior problems with it. It is a dye that makes the pictures clearer.

You will need to lie face down on a table. The table will have padded openings for your bare breasts. During the scan, the table will move slowly through a machine.

Lab tests
A pathologist is a doctor who's an expert in testing cells to find disease. He or she will test the tissue that was removed from your body. You may have had tissue removed from your breast, lymph nodes, or both.

Histologic typing
The pathologist will study the tissue samples using a microscope. If cancer is present, he or she will determine in which type of tissue it started. This is called histologic typing. Most breast cancers start in ductal cells.

Cancer grade
There are 3 grades of DCIS. Grade I looks the most like normal cells. It is the least likely to spread. Grade II also grows slowly. Grade III looks the least like normal cells. It is the most likely to spread. Grade III is often linked with comedo necrosis.

Comedo necrosis refers to the buildup of dead cells within the duct.

Estrogen receptor test
Estrogen is a hormone. Among some women, estrogen really helps the cancer cells grow. **See Figure 6**. The pathologist will test your cancer cells for estrogen receptors. Results are used to plan treatment.

IHC (**i**mmuno**h**isto**c**hemistry) is a lab test that detects hormone receptors. The pathologist will stain the cancer cells then view them with a microscope. He or she will assess how many cells have hormone receptors. Also, the amount of hormone receptors in the cells will be measured.

If at least 1 out of every 100 cancer cells have hormone receptors, the cancer is called hormone receptor–positive. Hormone receptor–negative breast cancer consists of fewer cells with hormone receptors. Hormone receptor–positive breast cancer often grows slower than hormone receptor–negative cancer.

Pathology report
All lab results are included in a pathology report. This report will be sent to your doctor. It is used to plan treatment.

There may be more than one report. Lab tests will be performed before treatment. More lab tests will be done if you have surgery.

Ask for a copy of each report. Your doctor will review the results with you. Take notes and ask questions.

Genetic counseling

Your disease or family history may suggest you have hereditary breast cancer. In this case, your doctor will refer you for genetic counseling. A genetic counselor is an expert in gene mutations that are related to disease. Your counselor can tell you more about your chances of having hereditary breast cancer.

Your counselor may suggest that you undergo genetic testing. *BRCA1* and *BRCA2* gene mutations are related to breast cancer. Other genes may be tested as well. Some genes may cause cancers other than just breast cancer. Your counselor will explain your test results and what to do next. Your test results may be used to guide treatment planning.

Some abnormal changes in genes, called VUS (**v**ariants of **u**nknown **s**ignificance), are not fully understood by doctors. Your doctors may know of research that aims to learn more. If interested, ask your doctors about taking part in such research.

Figure 6
Estrogen receptor–positive breast cancer

In some women, estrogen helps cancer cells grow. It enters cancer cells and attaches to receptors. The receptors then enter the nucleus and trigger cell growth.

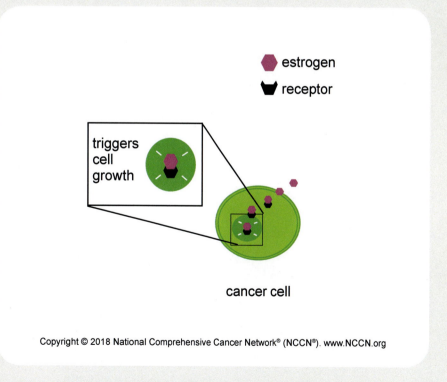

Copyright © 2018 National Comprehensive Cancer Network® (NCCN®). www.NCCN.org

Cancer treatment

The goal of treatment is to prevent DCIS from invading the stroma. Surgery is the central part of treatment. A list of treatment options is in **Guide 2**. You may have more than one option for treatment. Read Part 4 to learn some tips on making treatment decisions.

Lumpectomy + radiation therapy
A lumpectomy followed by radiation therapy is called breast-conserving therapy. It is an option for many but not all women with DCIS. Prior radiation, pregnancy, and certain health conditions may exclude this option.

A lumpectomy is a surgery that removes the tumor while sparing healthy tissue. **See Figure 7**. Some normal-looking tissue around the tumor's edge is also removed. This tissue is called a surgical margin.

Guide 2. Treatment for DCIS

What are the options?
• Lumpectomy + radiation therapy
• Total mastectomy ± sentinel lymph node biopsy
• Lumpectomy
• Clinical trial

**Figure 7
Lumpectomy**

A lumpectomy is a breast-conserving surgery. Your surgeon will make a cut into your breast large enough to remove the cancer. It will cause a small scar. There may be a dent in your breast that can be fixed with breast reconstruction.

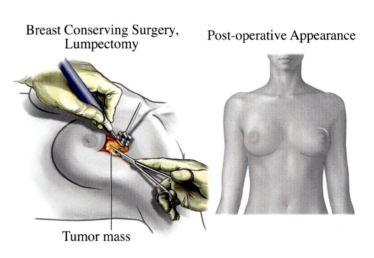

Breast Conserving Surgery, Lumpectomy

Post-operative Appearance

Tumor mass

Illustration Copyright © 2018 Nucleus Medical Media, All rights reserved. www.nucleusinc.com

3 Treatment guide: DCIS | Cancer treatment

Radiation therapy is given when the surgical margin is cancer-free. It treats cancer cells that may remain in the breast after lumpectomy. It uses high-energy x-rays to damage cancer cells. The cells either die or can't make new cancer cells.

Most of your breast will be treated with radiation. Whole breast radiation helps prevent the return of cancer in about half of women. Ask your doctor if your risk of the cancer coming back is low or high. If it's high, you may receive extra radiation called a boost.

Some women may receive radiation only to the lumpectomy site. This method is called partial breast irradiation. More research is needed on its outcomes. Ask your doctor if there's a clinical trial that you can join.

Total mastectomy ± sentinel lymph node biopsy

Some women with DCIS can't have a lumpectomy. It may not be an option because of your health. The tumor may be too large. Cancer may be found at the surgical margin. Your age might put you at risk for a second breast cancer.

Other women choose not to have a lumpectomy. Some women refuse because of how they want their breast to look after treatment. Others refuse because cancer can't return in a breast that's been removed. However, a second breast tumor can still occur in the other breast or in lymph nodes.

A total mastectomy is a surgery that removes the whole breast. **See Figure 8**. Chest muscle is not removed. This operation is also called a simple mastectomy. A skin-sparing mastectomy removes the breast but not the skin. Options for breast reconstruction are presented in Part 5.

Figure 8
Mastectomy

The whole breast is removed during a total mastectomy. An oval-shaped cut is often first made around the areola. The breast tissue is then detached and removed. You may have a draining tube for 2 or 3 weeks while you heal. A mastectomy causes a large scar.

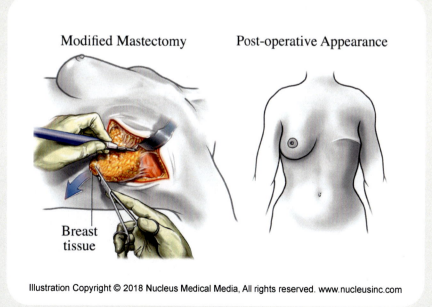

Illustration Copyright © 2018 Nucleus Medical Media, All rights reserved. www.nucleusinc.com

Before removing the breast, some lymph nodes may be removed. Sentinel nodes are the first nodes to which lymph travels after leaving the breast. An SLNB (**s**entinel **l**ymph **n**ode **b**iopsy) finds and removes 2 or 3 of these nodes. The nodes are then tested for cancer. Once the breast is removed, this biopsy can't be done. Instead, many lymph nodes would have to be removed to test for cancer.

Lumpectomy

Treatment with only a lumpectomy is an option for a small group of women. You must have a very low risk of the cancer coming back. So, the cancer must be very small and low grade. Surgical margins must be large and cancer-free. You should be 50 years of age or older. Ask your doctor if a lumpectomy alone is an option for you.

Clinical trial

A clinical trial is a type of research that studies a test or treatment in people. It gives people access to health care that otherwise can't usually be received. Ask your treatment team if there is an open clinical trial that you can join.

I sometimes wish that treatment wasn't such a bully... except when it comes to fighting the cancer.

– Lynn
Cancer Survivor

Risk-reduction treatment

Risk-reduction treatment may help prevent a second breast cancer. There are three main ways to reduce your risk. Talk with your doctor about which methods are right for you.

Lifestyle changes

Changes in your lifestyle may reduce your chance of a second breast cancer. Eating a more healthy diet may help. You might need to exercise more. You might need to achieve a healthy body weight. Ask your doctor for a lifestyle plan that is right for you.

Endocrine therapy

Endocrine therapy includes treatments that stop cancer growth caused by hormones. It is sometimes called hormone therapy. It is not the same as hormone replacement therapy.

Talk to your doctor about starting endocrine therapy. It may help prevent a second breast cancer if you had estrogen receptor–positive cancer. It is unknown how well endocrine therapy works if you had estrogen receptor–negative cancer. Your doctor may advise taking endocrine therapy based on other factors, such as family history.

There is more than one type of endocrine therapy. The type prescribed by doctors is partly based on if you have menstrual periods. Women who have menstrual periods receive tamoxifen. Women without menstrual periods receive tamoxifen or an aromatase inhibitor.

Endocrine therapy can cause side effects. These side effects include hot flashes, cataracts, leg cramps, joint pain, blood clots, and some cancers. Ask your treatment team for a complete list of side effects.

While taking endocrine therapy, you will have follow-up visits with your doctor. Tell your doctor about any new or worse symptoms. There may be ways to get relief. Some women will also need to get GYN (**gyn**ecologic) exams, vision tests, and bone density tests.

Surgery
A third risk-reduction treatment is surgery. A total mastectomy is an option to reduce your risk in a breast that did not have cancer. Options for breast reconstruction are presented in Part 5.

Your doctor may suggest that you have a bilateral salpingo-oophorectomy. This surgery removes both ovaries and both fallopian tubes. It is only advised if you have or very likely have mutations in the *BRCA1* and *BRCA2* genes.

Follow-up care

Follow-up care is important for your long-term health. It is started after treatment ends. There must be no signs or symptoms of cancer.

Medical history and physical exam
An update of your health history and physical exam are part of follow-up care. Both should be done every 6 to 12 months for 5 years. After 5 years of normal results, these tests are needed once a year.

Mammogram
A mammogram should be done every 12 months. The first one may be received as soon as 6 months after a breast-conserving treatment. Mammograms aren't needed if you had both breasts removed to reduce your cancer risk.

Review

- An exam and imaging of your breasts will be done to assess for abnormal tissue.

- A lab test is needed to test if the cancer is estrogen-receptor positive or negative.

- Genetic counseling can help assess if you have hereditary breast cancer.

- DCIS is treated with breast-conserving methods or a total mastectomy.

- Lifestyle changes, endocrine therapy, and surgery help to prevent future breast cancer.

- Follow-up care includes breast exams and mammograms.

4 Treatment guide: Breast reconstruction

29 Volume displacement
29 Implants & flaps
30 Nipple replacement
30 Review

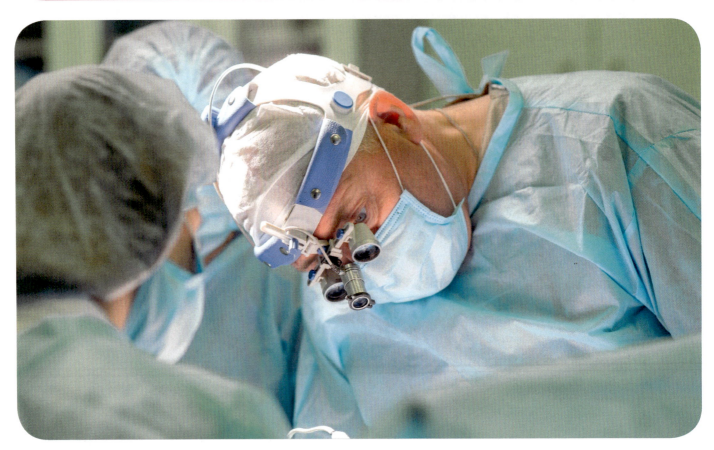

4 Treatment guide: Breast reconstruction — Volume displacement | Implants & flaps

After surgery, some women choose to have breast reconstruction. Other women use breast forms or do nothing. This chapter explains some details about breast reconstruction.

Volume displacement

If you will have a lumpectomy, your breast can be re-shaped. This procedure is called volume displacement. It is often done by the cancer surgeon right after the lumpectomy. He or she will shift the remaining breast tissue to fill the hole left by the removed tumor.

If volume displacement is planned, a larger piece of your breast will need to be removed. Despite a larger piece being removed, the natural look of your breast will be kept. Having a larger piece removed will likely reduce your chance of the cancer coming back.

You may not like the results of the volume displacement. In this case, breast revision surgery may help. This surgery is done by a plastic surgeon. A second volume displacement may be an option, too. A third option is to get breast implants or flaps, which are described next.

Implants & flaps

Breasts can be fully reconstructed with implants and flaps. All methods are generally safe, but as with any surgery, there are risks. Ask your treatment team for a complete list of side effects.

You may have a choice as to when breast reconstruction is done. Immediate reconstruction is finished within hours after removing the breast. Delayed reconstruction can occur months or years after the cancer surgery. A plastic surgeon performs breast reconstruction.

Implants

Breast implants are small bags filled with salt water, silicone gel, or both. **See Figure 9**. They are placed under the breast skin and muscle. A balloon-like device, called an expander, may be used first to stretch out tissue. It will be placed under your skin or muscle and enlarged every few weeks for two to three months.

Implants have a small risk of leaking. You may feel pain from the implant or expander. Scar tissue or tissue death occurs in some women.

**Figure 9
Breast implants**

Breast implants are one method of reconstructing breast. They are small bags filled with salt water, silicone gel, or both. They are placed under the breast skin and muscle. A balloon-like device, called an expander, may be used first to stretch out tissue.

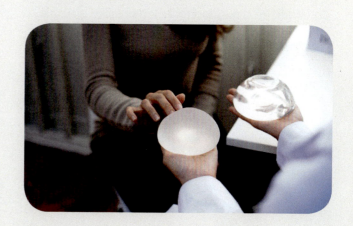

4 Treatment guide: Breast reconstruction | Nipple replacement | Review

Flaps

Breasts can be remade using tissue from your body, known as "flaps." Flaps are taken from the belly area, butt, or from under the shoulder blade. Some flaps are completely removed and then sewn in place. Other flaps stay attached but are slid over and sewn into place.

Flaps can cause problems. There may be tissue death. Death of fat cells may cause lumps. A hernia may occur from muscle weakness. Problems are more likely to occur among women who have diabetes or smoke.

Implants and flaps

Some breasts are reconstructed with both implants and flaps. This method may give the reconstructed breast more volume to match the other breast. For any reconstruction, you may need surgery on your real breast to match the two breasts in size and shape.

Nipple replacement

Like your breast, you can have your nipple remade. To rebuild a nipple, a plastic surgeon can use surrounding tissues. Also, nipples can be remade with tissue from the thigh, other nipple, or the sex organs between your legs (vulva). Tissue can be darkened with a tattoo to look more like a nipple.

Review

> Volume displacement is a shifting of the breast tissue to fill the hole left by a lumpectomy.

> Breasts that are fully removed can be remade with breast implants, flaps, or both.

> Removed nipples can be remade with body tissue.

5
Making treatment decisions

32 It's your choice
32 Questions to ask
37 Weighing your options
38 Websites
38 Review

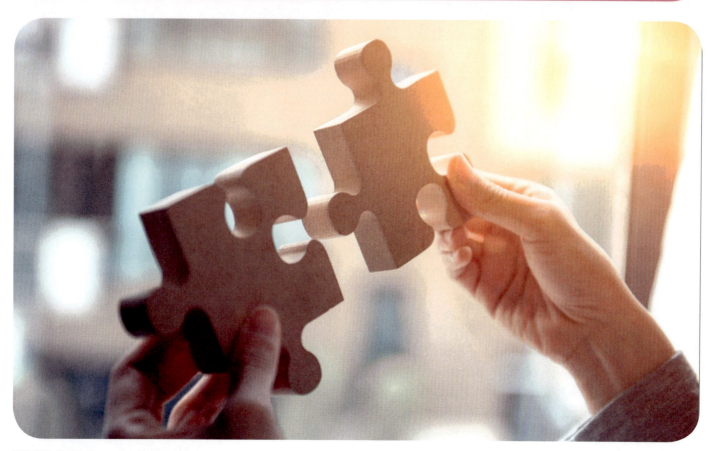

5 Making treatment decisions

It's your choice | Questions to ask

Having cancer is very stressful. While absorbing the fact that you have cancer, you have to learn about tests and treatments. In addition, the time you have to accept a treatment plan feels short. Parts 1 through 3 described breast cancer and treatment options. This chapter aims to help you make decisions that are in line with your beliefs, wishes, and values.

It's your choice

The role patients want in choosing their treatment differs. You may feel uneasy about making treatment decisions. This may be due to a high level of stress. It may be hard to hear or know what others are saying. Stress, pain, and drugs can limit your ability to make good decisions. You may feel uneasy because you don't know much about cancer. You've never heard the words used to describe cancer, tests, or treatments. Likewise, you may think that your judgment isn't any better than your doctors'.

Letting others decide which option is best may make you feel more at ease. But, whom do you want to make the decisions? You may rely on your doctors alone to make the right decisions. However, your doctors may not tell you which to choose if you have multiple good options. You can also have loved ones help. They can gather information, speak on your behalf, and share in decision-making with your doctors. Even if others decide which treatment you will receive, you still have to agree by signing a consent form.

On the other hand, you may want to take the lead or share in decision-making. Most patients do. In shared decision-making, you and your doctors share information, weigh the options, and agree on a treatment plan. Your doctors know the science behind your plan but you know your concerns and goals. By working together, you are likely to get a higher quality of care and be more satisfied. You'll likely get the treatment you want, at the place you want, and by the doctors you want.

Questions to ask

You may meet with experts from different fields of medicine. Strive to have helpful talks with each person. Prepare questions before your visit and ask questions if the person isn't clear. You can also record your talks and get copies of your medical records.

It may be helpful to have your spouse, partner, or a friend with you at these visits. A patient advocate or navigator might also be able to come. They can help to ask questions and remember what was said. Suggested questions to ask are listed on the following pages.

5 Making treatment decisions | Questions to ask

What's my diagnosis and prognosis?

It's important to know that there are different types of cancer. Cancer can greatly differ even when people have a tumor in the same organ. Based on your test results, your doctors can tell you which type of cancer you have. He or she can also give a prognosis. A prognosis is a prediction of the pattern and outcome of a disease. Knowing the prognosis may affect what you decide about treatment.

1. Where did the cancer start? In what type of cell? Is this cancer common?

2. Is this a fast- or slow-growing cancer?

3. What tests do you recommend for me?

4. Where will the tests take place? How long will the tests take and will any test hurt?

5. What if I am pregnant?

6. How do I prepare for testing?

7. Should I bring a list of my medications?

8. Should I bring someone with me?

9. How often are these tests wrong?

10. Would you give me a copy of the pathology report and other test results?

11. Who will talk with me about the next steps? When?

5 Making treatment decisions | Questions to ask

What are my options?

There is no single treatment practice that is best for all patients. There is often more than one treatment option along with clinical trial options. Your doctor will review your test results and recommend treatment options.

1. What will happen if I do nothing?

2. Can I just carefully monitor the cancer?

3. Do you consult NCCN recommendations when considering options?

4. Are you suggesting options other than what NCCN recommends? If yes, why?

5. Do your suggested options include clinical trials? Please explain why.

6. How do my age, health, and other factors affect my options? What if I am pregnant?

7. Which option is proven to work best?

8. Which options lack scientific proof?

9. What are the benefits of each option? Does any option offer a cure or long-term cancer control? Are my chances any better for one option than another? Less time-consuming? Less expensive?

10. What are the risks of each option? What are possible complications? What are the rare and common side effects? Short-lived and long-lasting side effects? Serious or mild side effects? Other risks?

11. How do you know if treatment is working?

12. What are my options if my treatment stops working?

13. What can be done to prevent or relieve the side effects of treatment?

5 Making treatment decisions | Questions to ask

What does each option require of me?

Many patients consider how each option will practically affect their lives. This information may be important because you have family, jobs, and other duties to take care of. You also may be concerned about getting the help you need. If you have more than one option, choosing the option that is the least taxing may be important to you.

1. Will I have to go to the hospital or elsewhere? How often? How long is each visit?

2. What do I need to think about if I will travel for treatment?

3. Do I have a choice of when to begin treatment? Can I choose the days and times of treatment?

4. How do I prepare for treatment? Do I have to stop taking any of my medicines? Are there foods I will have to avoid?

5. Should I bring someone with me when I get treated?

6. Will the treatment hurt?

7. How much will the treatment cost me? What does my insurance cover?

8. Will I miss work or school? Will I be able to drive?

9. Is home care after treatment needed? If yes, what type?

10. How soon will I be able to manage my own health?

11. When will I be able to return to my normal activities?

5 Making treatment decisions | Questions to ask

What is your experience?

More and more research is finding that patients treated by more experienced doctors have better results. It is important to learn if a doctor is an expert in the cancer treatment he or she is offering.

1. Are you board certified? If yes, in what area?

2. How many patients like me have you treated?

3. How many procedures like the one you're suggesting have you done?

4. Is this treatment a major part of your practice?

5. How many of your patients have had complications?

5 Making treatment decisions | Deciding between options

Deciding between options

Deciding which option is best can be hard. Doctors from different fields of medicine may have different opinions on which option is best for you. This can be very confusing. Your spouse or partner may disagree with which option you want. This can be stressful. In some cases, one option hasn't been shown to work better than another. Some ways to decide on treatment are discussed next.

2nd opinion

The time around a cancer diagnosis is very stressful. People with cancer often want to get treated as soon as possible. They want to make their cancer go away before it spreads farther. While cancer can't be ignored, there is time to think about and choose which option is best for you.

You may wish to have another doctor review your test results and suggest a treatment plan. This is called getting a 2nd opinion. You may completely trust your doctor, but a 2nd opinion on which option is best can help.

Copies of the pathology report, a DVD of the imaging tests, and other test results need to be sent to the doctor giving the 2nd opinion. Some people feel uneasy asking for copies from their doctors. However, a 2nd opinion is a normal part of cancer care.

When doctors have cancer, most will talk with more than one doctor before choosing their treatment. What's more, some health plans require a 2nd opinion. If your health plan doesn't cover the cost of a 2nd opinion, you have the choice of paying for it yourself.

If the two opinions are the same, you may feel more at peace about the treatment you accept to have. If the two opinions differ, think about getting a 3rd opinion. A 3rd opinion may help you decide between your options. Choosing your cancer treatment is a very important decision. It can affect your length and quality of life.

Decision aids

Decision aids are tools that help people make complex choices. For example, you may have to choose between two options that work equally as well. Sometimes making a decision is hard because there is a lack of science supporting a treatment.

Decision aids often focus on one decision point. In contrast, this book presents tests and treatment options for each point of care for women in general. Well-designed decision aids are based on research that identified what information people need to make decisions. They help you think about what's important based on your values and preferences.

A listing of decision aids can be found at decisionaid.ohri.ca/AZlist.html. Decision aids specific to early breast cancer are:

Genetic testing:
uofmhealth.org/health-library/zx3000

Breast-conserving therapy vs. mastectomy:
uofmhealth.org/health-library/tv6530#zx3718

Breast reconstruction after mastectomy:
uofmhealth.org/health-library/tb1934#zx3672

Support groups

Besides talking to health experts, it may help to talk to patients who have walked in your shoes. Support groups often consist of people at different stages of treatment. Some may be in the process of deciding while others may be finished with treatment. At support groups, you can ask questions and hear about the experiences of other people with breast cancer.

5 Making treatment decisions | Websites | Review

Compare benefits and downsides

Every option has benefits and downsides. Consider these when deciding which option is best for you. Talking to others can help identify benefits and downsides you haven't thought of. Scoring each factor from 0 to 10 can also help since some factors may be more important to you than others.

Websites

American Cancer Society
cancer.org/cancer/breast-cancer.html

Breast Cancer Alliance
breastcanceralliance.org

Breastcancer.org
breastcancer.org

FORCE: Facing Our Risk of Cancer Empowered
facingourrisk.org

Living Beyond Breast Cancer (LBBC)
lbbc.org

National Cancer Institute (NCI)
cancer.gov/types/breast

NCCN for Patients®
nccn.org/patients

Sharsheret
sharsheret.org

Young Survival Coalition (YSC)
youngsurvival.org

Review

> Shared decision-making is a process in which you and your doctors plan treatment together.

> Asking your doctors questions is vital to getting the information you need to make informed decisions.

> Getting a 2nd opinion, using decision aids, attending support groups, and comparing benefits and downsides may help you decide which treatment is best for you.

Glossary

40 Dictionary

42 Acronyms

Dictionary

areola
A darker, round area of skin on the breast around the nipple.

aromatase inhibitor
A drug that lowers the level of estrogen in the body.

bilateral salpingo-oophorectomy
Surgery that removes both ovaries and both fallopian tubes.

biopsy
A procedure that removes fluid or tissue samples to be tested for a disease.

boost
An extra dose of radiation to a specific area of the body.

breast-conserving therapy
A cancer treatment that includes removing a breast lump and radiation therapy.

breast implant
A small bag filled with salt water, gel, or both that is used to remake breasts.

breast reconstruction
An operation that creates new breasts.

cancer stage
A rating of the outlook of a cancer based on its growth and spread.

carcinoma
A cancer of cells that line the inner or outer surfaces of the body.

carcinoma in situ
A cancer that has not grown into tissue that would allow it to spread.

clinical breast exam
Touching of a breast by a health expert to feel for diseases.

clinical trial
A type of research that assesses health tests or treatments.

connective tissue
Supporting and binding tissue that surrounds other tissues and organs.

contrast
A dye put into your body to make clearer pictures during imaging tests.

core needle biopsy
A procedure that removes tissue samples with a hollow needle. Also called core biopsy.

diagnostic bilateral mammogram
Pictures of the insides of both breasts that are made from a set of x-rays.

duct
A tube-shaped structure through which milk travels to the nipple.

ductal carcinoma in situ (DCIS)
A breast cancer that has not grown outside the breast ducts.

endocrine therapy
A cancer treatment that stops the making or action of estrogen. Also called hormone therapy.

estrogen
A hormone that causes female body traits.

estrogen receptor
A protein inside of cells that binds to estrogen.

estrogen receptor–negative
A type of breast cancer that doesn't use estrogen to grow.

estrogen receptor–positive
A type of breast cancer that uses estrogen to grow.

gene
Coded instructions in cells for making new cells and controlling how cells behave.

genetic counseling
Expert guidance on the chance for a disease that is passed down in families.

hereditary breast cancer
Breast cancer that was likely caused by abnormal genes passed down from parent to child.

hormone
A chemical in the body that triggers a response from cells or organs.

Dictionary

immunohistochemistry (IHC)
A lab test of cancer cells to find specific cell traits involved in abnormal cell growth.

invasive breast cancer
The growth of breast cancer into the breast's supporting tissue (stroma).

lobular carcinoma in situ (LCIS)
A health condition of abnormal cells within the breast's milk-making gland.

lobule
A gland in the breast that makes breast milk.

lumpectomy
An operation that removes a small breast cancer tumor.

lymph
A clear fluid containing white blood cells.

lymph node
A small, bean-shaped disease-fighting structure.

magnetic resonance imaging (MRI)
A test that uses radio waves and powerful magnets to make pictures of the insides of the body.

mammogram
A picture of the insides of the breast that is made by an x-ray test.

mastectomy
An operation that removes the whole breast.

medical history
A report of all your health events and medications.

mutation
An abnormal change.

noninvasive breast cancer
Breast cancer that has not grown into tissue from which it can spread.

partial breast irradiation
Treatment with radiation that is received at the site of the removed breast tumor.

pathologist
A doctor who's an expert in testing cells and tissue to find disease.

physical exam
A study of the body by a health expert for signs of disease.

primary tumor
The first mass of cancer cells.

radiation therapy
A treatment that uses high-energy rays.

risk-reduction treatment
Methods that aim to lessen the chance of getting a disease.

sentinel lymph node
The first lymph node to which cancer cells spread after leaving a tumor.

sentinel lymph node biopsy (SLNB)
An operation to remove the disease-fighting structures (lymph nodes) to which cancer first spreads. Also called sentinel lymph node dissection.

side effect
An unhealthy or unpleasant physical or emotional response to treatment.

skin-sparing mastectomy
An operation that removes all breast tissue but saves as much breast skin as possible.

stroma
A type of body tissue that supports and connects other tissue.

surgical margin
The normal-looking tissue around a tumor that was removed during an operation.

total mastectomy
An operation that removes the entire breast but no chest muscles. Also called simple mastectomy.

ultrasound
A test that uses sound waves to take pictures of the inside of the body.

vulva
The outer female organs that are between the legs.

whole breast radiation
Treatment with radiation of the entire breast.

Acronyms

AJCC
American Joint Committee on Cancer

DCIS
ductal carcinoma in situ

DNA
deoxyribonucleic acid

GYN
gynecologic

IHC
immunohistochemistry

LCIS
lobular carcinoma in situ

MRI
magnetic resonance imaging

SLNB
sentinel lymph node biopsy

VUS
variants of unknown significance

NCCN Panel Members

NCCN Panel Members for Breast Cancer

William J. Gradishar, MD/Chair
Robert H. Lurie Comprehensive Cancer Center of Northwestern University

Benjamin O. Anderson, MD/Vice-Chair
Fred Hutchinson Cancer Research Center/Seattle Cancer Care Alliance

Rebecca Aft, MD, PhD
Siteman Cancer Center at Barnes-Jewish Hospital and Washington University School of Medicine

Ron Balassanian, MD
UCSF Helen Diller Family Comprehensive Cancer Center

Sarah L. Blair, MD
UC San Diego Moores Cancer Center

Harold J. Burstein, MD, PhD
Dana-Farber/Brigham and Women's Cancer Center

*Amy Cyr, MD
Siteman Cancer Center at Barnes-Jewish Hospital and Washington University School of Medicine

Chau Dang, MD
Memorial Sloan Kettering Cancer Center

Anthony D. Elias, MD
University of Colorado Cancer Center

William B. Farrar, MD
The Ohio State University Comprehensive Cancer Center - James Cancer Hospital and Solove Research Institute

Andres Forero, MD
University of Alabama at Birmingham Comprehensive Cancer Center

Sharon H. Giordano, MD, MPH
The University of Texas MD Anderson Cancer Center

Matthew Goetz, MD
Mayo Clinic Cancer Center

Lori J. Goldstein, MD
Fox Chase Cancer Center

Steven J. Isakoff, MD, PhD
Massachusetts General Hospital Cancer Center

Janice Lyons, MD
Case Comprehensive Cancer Center/University Hospitals Seidman Cancer Center and Cleveland Clinic Taussig Cancer Institute

P. Kelly Marcom, MD
Duke Cancer Institute

Ingrid A. Mayer, MD
Vanderbilt-Ingram Cancer Center

Beryl McCormick, MD
Memorial Sloan Kettering Cancer Center

Meena S. Moran, MD
Yale Cancer Center/Smilow Cancer Hospital

Ruth M. O'Regan, MD
University of Wisconsin Carbone Cancer Center

Sameer A. Patel, MD
Fox Chase Cancer Center

Lori J. Pierce, MD
University of Michigan Rogel Cancer Center

Elizabeth C. Reed, MD
Fred & Pamela Buffett Cancer Center

Lee S. Schwartzberg, MD
St. Jude Children's Research Hospital/The University of Tennessee Health Science Center

Amy Sitapati, MD
UC San Diego Moores Cancer Center

Karen Lisa Smith, MD, MPH
The Sidney Kimmel Comprehensive Cancer Center at Johns Hopkins

Mary Lou Smith, JD, MBA
Patient Advocate
Research Advocacy Network

Hatem Soliman, MD
Moffitt Cancer Center

George Somlo, MD
City of Hope Comprehensive Cancer Center

Melinda L. Telli, MD
Stanford Cancer Institute

John H. Ward, MD
Huntsman Cancer Institute at the University of Utah

NCCN Staff

Dorothy A. Shead, MS
Director, Patient Information Operations

Rashmi Kumar, PhD
Director, Clinical Information Operations

* Reviewed the clinical content of this book.
For disclosures, visit www.nccn.org/about/disclosure.aspx.

NCCN Member Institutions

Fred & Pamela Buffett Cancer Center
Omaha, Nebraska
800.999.5465
nebraskamed.com/cancer

Case Comprehensive Cancer Center/ University Hospitals Seidman Cancer Center and Cleveland Clinic Taussig Cancer Institute
Cleveland, Ohio
800.641.2422 • UH Seidman Cancer Center
uhhospitals.org/seidman
866.223.8100 • CC Taussig Cancer Institute
my.clevelandclinic.org/services/cancer
216.844.8797 • Case CCC
case.edu/cancer

City of Hope Comprehensive Cancer Center
Los Angeles, California
800.826.4673
cityofhope.org

Dana-Farber/Brigham and Women's Cancer Center Massachusetts General Hospital Cancer Center
Boston, Massachusetts
877.332.4294
dfbwcc.org
massgeneral.org/cancer

Duke Cancer Institute
Durham, North Carolina
888.275.3853
dukecancerinstitute.org

Fox Chase Cancer Center
Philadelphia, Pennsylvania
888.369.2427
foxchase.org

Huntsman Cancer Institute at the University of Utah
Salt Lake City, Utah
877.585.0303
huntsmancancer.org

Fred Hutchinson Cancer Research Center/Seattle Cancer Care Alliance
Seattle, Washington
206.288.7222 • seattlecca.org
206.667.5000 • fredhutch.org

The Sidney Kimmel Comprehensive Cancer Center at Johns Hopkins
Baltimore, Maryland
410.955.8964
hopkinskimmelcancercenter.org

Robert H. Lurie Comprehensive Cancer Center of Northwestern University
Chicago, Illinois
866.587.4322
cancer.northwestern.edu

Mayo Clinic Cancer Center
Phoenix/Scottsdale, Arizona
Jacksonville, Florida
Rochester, Minnesota
800.446.2279 • Arizona
904.953.0853 • Florida
507.538.3270 • Minnesota
mayoclinic.org/departments-centers/mayo-clinic-cancer-center

Memorial Sloan Kettering Cancer Center
New York, New York
800.525.2225
mskcc.org

Moffitt Cancer Center
Tampa, Florida
800.456.3434
moffitt.org

The Ohio State University Comprehensive Cancer Center - James Cancer Hospital and Solove Research Institute
Columbus, Ohio
800.293.5066
cancer.osu.edu

Roswell Park Comprehensive Cancer Center
Buffalo, New York
877.275.7724
roswellpark.org

Siteman Cancer Center at Barnes-Jewish Hospital and Washington University School of Medicine
St. Louis, Missouri
800.600.3606
siteman.wustl.edu

St. Jude Children's Research Hospital The University of Tennessee Health Science Center
Memphis, Tennessee
888.226.4343 • stjude.org
901.683.0055 • westclinic.com

Stanford Cancer Institute
Stanford, California
877.668.7535
cancer.stanford.edu

University of Alabama at Birmingham Comprehensive Cancer Center
Birmingham, Alabama
800.822.0933
www3.ccc.uab.edu

UC San Diego Moores Cancer Center
La Jolla, California
858.657.7000
cancer.ucsd.edu

UCSF Helen Diller Family Comprehensive Cancer Center
San Francisco, California
800.689.8273
cancer.ucsf.edu

University of Colorado Cancer Center
Aurora, Colorado
720.848.0300
coloradocancercenter.org

University of Michigan Rogel Cancer Center
Ann Arbor, Michigan
800.865.1125
mcancer.org

The University of Texas MD Anderson Cancer Center
Houston, Texas
800.392.1611
mdanderson.org

University of Wisconsin Carbone Cancer Center
Madison, Wisconsin
608.265.1700
uwhealth.org/cancer

Vanderbilt-Ingram Cancer Center
Nashville, Tennessee
800.811.8480
vicc.org

Yale Cancer Center/ Smilow Cancer Hospital
New Haven, Connecticut
855.4.SMILOW
yalecancercenter.org

Notes

Index

2nd opinion 37

biopsy 17, 18, 24–26

breast reconstruction 24–25, 27–29, 37

carcinoma in situ 12–13, 18, 20–27

clinical breast exam 6, 19, 21

clinical trial 18, 24–26, 34

genetic counseling 23, 27

endocrine therapy 26, 27

estrogen receptor 22–23, 26

immunohistochemistry (IHC) 22

lumpectomy 18, 24–26, 29–30

lymph 8–10, 13, 18, 26

magnetic resonance imaging (MRI) 16, 22

mammogram 16–17, 19, 21–22, 27

mastectomy 18, 24–25, 27, 37

medical history 19, 21, 27

NCCN Member Institutions 44

NCCN Panel Members 43

nipple replacement 30

physical exam 19, 21, 27

radiation therapy 18–19, 24–25

risk reduction 18

salpingo-oophorectomy 27

sentinel lymph node biopsy (SLNB) 18, 24–26

Horsham Township Library

Made in the USA
Middletown, DE
19 February 2019